A Break from the Chaos

Part 2

By T.L. Larson

For my father.

The strongest man I ever knew.

You showed me the meaning of true strength.

Physically, mentally, spiritually.

You are so deeply missed.

A Break from the Chaos: Part 2

A Healthy Nugget book.

Cover by Ariane Larson.

For permissions contact:
Abreakfromthechaos@gmail.com

ISBN: 978-1-7362955-1-9

A Break from the Chaos: Part 2

A Healthy Nugget book.

Cover by Ariane Larson.

For permissions contact:
Abreakfromthechaos@gmail.com

ISBN: 978-1-7362955-1-9

For my father.

The strongest man I ever knew.

You showed me the meaning of true strength.

Physically, mentally, spiritually.

You are so deeply missed.

Table of Contents

Table of Contents

Table of Contents

Preface

So you're back for more...

Welcome!

I wish I could tell you all has been rainbows and unicorns, which unsurprisingly with 2 little girls in my life now, there is indeed more rainbows and unicorns than before. However, it has been a tough few years. A *very* tough few years.

Starting practice in the midst of a global pandemic sure had its challenges, but nothing could prepare us for losing dad to COVID-19 on December 25th of 2020. Never have I felt so impacted by a single life event. To this day nearly 3 years out, I still can't seem to get over his loss. He is missed so dearly. He was such a light in our lives. A light in so many people's lives. Without him, the world is indeed darker.

But there is always room for more light in this world.

Our family has been blessed with 2 little girls that now seem to run our household. They somehow seem to occupy 99.9% of our free time (and a good bit of our sleep time).
So therefore, what I thought I could accomplish in another year, (in finishing part 2 of this series), took 3 years instead! So by my calculations, part 3 should be finished in approximately 9 years. So, sorry for my eager fan(s) out there. Don't hold your breath for the next round.

I more and more believe those who say time flies. I now fear I may blink and a few more years will have flown by. I envy the days when I was a child, when 10 minutes felt like an eternity.

Now looking back at my time in medicine, (several years as a premed student, 4 years as a medical student, 3 years in family medicine residency and now approaching 4 years in practice) I can't help but feel that I have only just started yesterday, but also feel like I have been doing this for eternity.

As time passes, people move on, little girls grow bigger, and early speckles of grey begin to find their way onto my scalp. Someone please invent a time machine soon! I often wish I could bring this moving train to a halt, but it is too strong and keeps barreling forward.

If you have this book in front of you, thank you.

Thank you for making my words come to life ever so slightly more. I enjoy sharing these thoughts and words with you. I hope that you will find something from them once again. A connection, a deeper meaning, enjoyment, tears of sorrow, tears of joy. Or perhaps thoughts that whoever is writing this, is just a little crazy. That's ok! I think all of us doctors are probably a little crazy. I mean, who would willingly sign up for a minimum of 11 years of hard work, free/cheap labor, and endless studying to only drive yourself further and further into debt?!

These scribbles and poems are a collection of patient encounters, struggles with loss, joys of life, and of course a few random things that have no bearing on anything at all. Perhaps even a spooky tale or two.

Once again, reader beware! Not too many happily-ever after tales in here. But I think there is a little something for everyone here.

I hope you do enjoy!

Best wishes and happy reading.

A return to the Chaos.

51

The Pen

No longer willed to write
Worn down by time and hardship
After many hours of long talks
Moments of thought
The pen asked for a moment of respite

After much coercion
The pen emerged from slumber
Only the ink had dried at its tip
It scratched fervently on parchment
Yielding mere bits of markings

After scratching an old itch
The ink began to flow
The pen stuttered, muttered, and fluttered about
Too many pauses and ink blots clouded the page
Will it ever be the same?

Like old muscles that need tuning
The hand started pruning
Traversing the paper, to get others swooning
The pen had returned
Only to find itself out of ink.

52

The Blank Page

The blank page
so empty
stares back taunting

Void

The blank page
so bright
urges to be fulfilled

Unrealized

53

Hangers

Sometimes I walk into the closet
With no other purpose
Than to turn hangers the wrong way
My own rebellion to your order

Turning some the wrong way
I know you will notice
And I will laugh

One collar kisses another
Instead of marching in formation
Disobeying instruction
Inconceivable

A blue shirt slides in to the reds
And I'm grinning
Knowing the scolding that will come

54

Gravity

Gravity
Strong, stable, steady
Stands by devoted
Keeps one upright

Feet beneath, on firm ground
Keeps one from flying too high
Keeps dreams in check
Rooted in reality

Gravity
Stubborn, steadfast, staunch
Struggle to break free
Keeps us subdued

Pulls us down, holds us back
Keeps us from reaching too high
Keeps us from the heavens
Limits our potential

55

The Next Act

Forward facing
Just stopped pacing
Can't keep the heart from racing

Breathing rushed
Face is flushed
Bearing the weight to keep from crushed

A deep, deep sigh
As I say goodbye
To some final thoughts of the one before

Knock

Smile in place

Greet the next one I face

Never will you know the trials laid before

The widowed mother
The depressed brother
The dying man and his greatest fan

But for the next 10 minutes, you and me
Together our greatest concern will be...

Your stubbed toe.

Beat down the Chaos.

6

I Will Not be Beat!

Let's jump back to the early 1980s for story time.

A roaring crowd filled the stadium. The crowd composed mostly with young men, and some old. Most were more than a few beers in. They all sat around waiting to watch a few good fights. Most too afraid to enter the ring themselves, as only the biggest, toughest, strongest entered this ring.

The ring and ropes rested comfortably in the center. The canvas already wet with sweat and already stained with scattered drops of fresh blood, haphazardly wiped from its surface.

The Tri-State Tough Man Competition was underway…

One of these brave men competing was none other than Jeff Larson, commonly known by his friends as "Lars." For better or worse, by the time he reached his 20's, he was no stranger to fighting. He had been in plenty of fights before. Though not out of malice, as Lars was kind spirited, and he had seldom ventured on in competition. Fights became a regular occurrence growing up with 2 brothers; who he both fought with and fought to protect. Needless to say, he had been in a fair share of fights. But today was different… There were no family, friends, or school yard rivals he would be fighting today. There were also no weight classes to prevent the giants from attempting to squash the little, and there were notably some "biggins" signed up. Even though at 6 foot tall, Lars was no "tiny," he was by no means the biggest. This didn't bother him one bit. You see, Lars had a motto, and he stuck by it. Put simply...

"I will not be beat."

And for several matches this held true.

All the way up to the final match.

He made it to the championship fight, hardly breaking a sweat... Well, I'll take that back. Dad was a known "sweater". Known to soak completely through his workout outfits. And I mean dripping, wet. He most likely was drenched in sweat! But he hardly had a scratch on him. Taking out several competitors with ease, he cruised to the championship match.

His final match arrived and his competitor was a beast. A ginormous beast at that. Again, there were no weight classes. And while one may say, "it's not the size of the dog in the fight..." Size can definitely account for something.

Dave Rusch recounts thinking at the time, *"Oh boy, Jeff's in trouble here."*

But once again, Jeff Larson walked out to this ring for the final fight, without a glimpse of fear. He frequently brought up the concept and was a firm believer of "mind over matter."

"I will not be beat!"

The fighters approached each other. Fire burned in each of the competitors' eyes. Not only was the title on the line, but a little extra cash never hurt either. As a hungry college kid, some extra cash sure makes victory a good bit sweeter.

Fists touched and the match was on.

The crowd was getting settled for a good one, but it quickly erupted. The crowd roared to life after only the first two punches.

Jeff Larson stood proud and strong over his goliath, now lying dazed on the canvas. Two punches into the final fight and a new champion was crowned.

Turns out, the "*size of the fight in the dog*" probably does indeed make a bigger difference.

Word spread quickly around town of the evening's results. When Jeff Larson walked in to an establishment, heads turned. Respect he had won.

Dave Rusch recalls a little victory celebration after the tournament. *"After the big match, Lars said 'Ruschy, get your best on and we are going out.' We did just that. We went to a high-end restaurant with 3-piece suits, cowboy hats, and cigars. The drink of the night…Whiskey. People would ask us what we were celebrating as we enjoyed our steak and lobster. Our story was: we just hit it big on our oil rigs in Texas."*

57

Unbeaten

You can bring your best
You can bring your worst
Make the weather hot
Make the weather cold
Rain, snow, sleet, ice
A hurricane will suffice

The one thing you will have to consider
Is that...

“I will not be beat.”

58

Sunny Disposition

Your smile so innocent
Could lighten anyone's day

Small
Vulnerable
Fragile

Yet, you fear so little
Especially in the arms of others

Each day you grow a little more
Learn a little more
Move a little more.

Nothing could falter
Your sunny disposition

59

What is Faith

God is good
God is great
So *why* would one hesitate?

Debate, debate, deliberate

What is faith without doubt
Climb to the mountain and shout your vies
But who will hear your desolate cries
As more and more fears arise

Questions here and there, and everywhere

Have *the* no faith??

For He will
show ye thine path.

60

Little Ones

The yard is unkept, but the house is clean
Aside from little toys that litter once pristine floors.
Sisyphus may have had it easy

Well lived in, by little feet that pitter and patter
Why bother painting the smudges made today
Crayons tomorrow will cover them enough

Thank goodness for mama
Who stays sane
Who stays sane despite your sustained silliness

Life changes

in an instant.

61

Waiting for You

One day
You were already gone

I used your tools
I cleaned your gear
I read your books
I sat with your dog

We waited

Waited for you to come home
Waited for life to move on

62

Cooking for One

It's hard to cook for one.

So dependent at first.
Wishing for cookies and fried chicken
Forced to eat broccoli

Time brings departure
A brief moment fending for self
Plenty of meals burnt

Too little, too much
It's hard to cook for one's self

Partnered up
One meal becomes two
Quickly grows to more

Dinnerware worn
Plates begin to break
No longer needing to be replaced

A plate is plenty
But it's hard to cook for one.

63

A Wishful Greeting

You'd be happy to know
Your dog stays true
Fur greyed with time
She approaches, thinking I'm you

Cataracts dull her once sharp eyes
Little more than shadows now
A cold wet nose
She sniffs at our greeting

Her tail wags
Droops slightly
Still happy to see me
Disappointed, I'm not you

64

Flowers

When you left

Flowers came

They withered

Too quickly

Then they left too

65

Captive

Been stressed

Depressed

In some state of duress

Held prisoner in this state.

A word can change everything.

66

Helpless

Helpless is how I would describe you
Sitting cross-legged in your oversized sweater
My regular sized sweater
In fact, once his sweater

Sitting there anxious
We talk of the weather
It has been cold weather
Hard to say whether…

Realization
What little control we have

Tissues in hand
Tears coat you
Tears not for you
Tears shed for him

Nothing to do
But pray.

67
Wounded

Wounded
I am uncertain how to heal
feeling weaker as the tears pour out
You were our strength
Our leader
Our teacher
Father

Wounded
I am certain this wound won't heal
But they say it gets better with time
I doubt them
This hole will never be filled
Your presence too large
Solid

Wounded
I believe I am starting to heal
Feeling stronger as the path becomes more clear
Learning to teach
A small new addition
Brings so much
hope

You would adore her

68

Imagine

It's so hard not to imagine

The What if's
The Could have been's
The Would be's

If only...

69

Grateful

I am grateful
For the times we had
And the times we would have had

I can picture our adventures
Paths of old
And those never taken

I am grateful
For the legacy you left
The legacy we will continue

I am grateful
You didn't have to grow old
You went out strong
Never having to see your own body wither

I am grateful
For the love you gave
And the love you left

I am grateful
For the life you lived
The life you made
And the lives you made live

Dad,
I am so grateful for you.

70

Unconditional

The pain I felt from loss
~~Is insurmountable~~
~~Has been insurmountable~~
I thought was insurmountable

Then you came into this world.
The love and joy I feel for you
Little girl
Is truly insurmountable

Chaos reigns king.

71

Foolishly Fixing

You came to me with problems I could not fix
Though I did not realize at the time

We changed your medicines
We took your blood
We ran our tests

Family demanded we fix you
Foolish, I tried.

If only we had opened our eyes
To look at your limited future

Decline inevitable
Already had begun
Unable to stop the inertia

Foolish, I tried.

72

Alone

Home alone, at night
Too quiet, the world shuts down tight
Lights out, time for rest
One last check, secure the nest

No daylight left

Creeping bereft

Back door locked
Windows shut tight
Before lie down tonight
The front door...

The padlock there
But the handle down there....

A knock at the door

But there's no one there

The door knob twists

But there's no one there

Heart sinks
Head swims

Dare to look out there
Where… there is no one there?

Wind picks up
Windows rattle
A whisper creeps
"Let me in"

But… there's nobody there

Eyes closed tight
Dark as night
Closed off ears
World gets quiet

Because…
There's nobody there.

73

These Monsters are Real

They walk upright

keep you up at night.

They plant seeds of doubt

hold in your shout.

They look back at you in the mirror

but they are nothing to fear…

Are they nothing to fear?

74

Those Haunting Eyes

Those haunting eyes I still see

Wide eyed
Quick in breath

In utter complete distress

Hurry, hurry
I hear death

Fix me.

75

Belly of the Beast

Should I have known
What lay inside your belly
Was more insidious than we could have imagined
I would have acted sooner

When you came to me yellow
My heart sunk
I think we all knew, but wouldn't believe
Until the scans sealed your fate

Placebo Effect

76

When Life Gives You Lemons

When life gives you lemons
You may find all the sugar is gone

When you finally find some sugar
You may find the lemons have gone rotten

When you decide to plant the seeds
You may find the soil is too hard and dry

When life gives you lemons
You may find it's better to just buy the lemonade

77

Tech Knowledgey

Darkness is extinguished by the glow of screens as we find our way,
In a world where knowledge flows from fingertips without delay,
amidst this digital tide we swoon and sway,
To a future where minds begin to fray.

As more algorithms guide the choices we make,
Our critical thinking begins to quake,
As technology's grip tightens and starts to take,
The human intellect will slowly break

In search of answers, we swipe and click,
deep understanding grows ever slick,
Our quest for wisdom begins to stick,
As shallow information hides the trick.

In a world where technology is so often sought,
Lest not forget the value of thought.

78
Blind to Time

Losing vision
Losing sight
Each day quickly turns to night

Days blur
Evenings fly
How and why does time pass by?

So much to do
So much to see
Quickly….

79

Comfort Zone

Nature's call, still ignored
In air cooled fridges we are stored
world outside, we seldom roam
comfort keeps us close to home.

Amidst modern comfort's tight embrace
We drift through life at easy pace.
In seeking ease, we may forget
Life brings challenge, we should not regret.

Nature's bounty, we rarely eat.
Food too processed, in wrappers neat.
Screens and couches, we found our zone
In spite of health, we now postpone

Convenience reigns king, health forego
In chase of comfort, we grow... Grow... Grow

80

The Last Piece

A meal so tasty
all eyes dance around the last piece.

A taste so heavenly
all are insatiable.

Golden crust, crisp.
Praised by scattered kneeling crumbs
that could never live up to the whole.

Self improvement, Self destruction

81
Waking Up to A

When I wake up tomorrow
Will I be…
Agitated
Angry
Annoyed
Anxious
Apathetic
Asleep?

When I wake up tomorrow
I hope I will be…
Accomplished
Adapted
Affectionate
Amiable
Attentive
Alive?

82

OCPD

Hours utilized and wasted
As you've revised and basted
Pouring your heart and soul
Into a simple irrelevant task

Explicitly meticulous
Complicitly ridiculous
Stuck in your own captivity
intense attention to detail

Inflexible in concern
Unfixable you spurn
No one else cares
Yet the work continues

This labor of love?
Indefinitely unfinished

83

Comfort Kills

Modern life
comfort found
ease we chase
Where's our grace?
Bright light screens
Their glowing light
entice us with endless night
We sit still
bodies waste
deep desires soon misplaced
The chair, the couch
They hold us down
comfort's grip
muscles rip
bones grow frail,
In stagnation, we will fail.

84

O Phobia! My Phobia!

What plagues thee so dear?

Fear of clowns
Fear of frowns
How to turn them upside downs

Fear of spiders
Fear of lighters
Please no more of these all nighters

Fear of heights
Fear of bites
Intergalactic Troglodytes?

Fear of tears
Fear of spears
Perhaps we're in too many beers!

85

Full Moon

The walls are grey
The floor is grey
The ceiling... grey
Even the clouds are grey, floating just outside

There's a full moon tonight
Addiction precedes affliction

Red rivers flow to the floor
Splatters the walls
Scrapes the ceiling
Can't quite reach the clouds

Darkness falls
Despite the moon's glow

The walls are black
The floor is black
The ceiling... black
Even the clouds are black, hovering loosely inside

Reluctant to change
Even as the sun begins to rise

The walls turned blue
How do you do?
Saw the sky melt
How have you felt?

Talked to dead friends
Never quite made amends
Rolled in blood
Just before the flood

Wounds still ache
Unable to catch a break
Consuming poison to distort reality
Brought back down to some form of gravity

The floor is green
Life sure is mean.
The ceiling is peeling
Let's start the healing.

The walls are white
The floor is white
The ceiling... white
Even the clouds are white, soaring through clear skies

Just in time for another full moon.

Thinking in circles

86

Shower Thoughts

Sometimes the best ideas come in the shower
Oh thy words have such great power

Thoughts and ideas, such grand intuition

But why, oh why?
By the last drop dry

Do these ideas never come to fruition?

87

The Hands of Time

A faint, blue river heads north
Traveling through a pale, white barren landscape

The veiny river soon enters a valley
Nestled between two enlarging calcified mountains

The digit extends along an overgrown rocky shore
Unyielding and refusing to be remolded

Turning the earth's crust over reveals cracks
Present from the beginning, deepened with time

Following crevices south approaches a radiant drumbeat
Ensuring the life blood within.

88

What to Value?

Money most certainly grows on trees
if you know which ones to plant

Those trees will grow and yield fruit in time
If you have the luxury to wait

Time however, is the most valuable currency
And who has time to waste?

89

Seats

My office chair is much too worn
Squeaking and complaining of the weight it bears

My sofa cushion is much too stiff
Always inviting, but so little time to break it in

90

Weathered Faith

Old pine narrow, dry
Weathered oak strong hearty wide
South wind, soon subsides

Life is but a dream.

91

Stare

Do you know what color your eyes are
What color they really are??

Can you even look yourself in the eyes

Can you see the fire
Or was it put out
Was it ever lit

Does anyone look back

Does anyone see

Can you see??

92

Baby Snuggles

My chest is your pillow
A perfect fit
I already miss each day past

A Wish for time to stand still
But I know if it did
You'd cease to grow

So keep on growing and learning
As cruel time keeps turning
I wish the world for you

But how I wish these moments lasted forever

93
Fever Dream

When I was a child, sick with fever
I saw soldiers marching on the ceiling
I chased giant frogs in the living room
I stood paralyzed in the dark hallway
Afraid of what was in front of me
Afraid of what was behind me

94

Sunrise to Sunset

Filled with longing and mirth
admiration, adoration
when I see you.
Curious and energized
no other could match
no other except, maybe that of another toddler.
Each day competition begins,
a question is asked,
who will crash first, by last light?
You win more frequent than one might expect.
Some would think it too much,
but we'd have it no other way
as you fill us with so much longing and mirth.

95

Dreams

If I am lucky, as I lay down
I may be treated to a trip uptown

Where whimsical wonderlands come to reality
Where beautiful landscapes are without calamity

Dreams, oh lovely dreams
I now have the strength to climb a tree
Power of might, power of flight
Skills I simply wish, come to be

Cobblestone streets pave the way
Golden lights brighten the day

Warmth of company
Laughing with friends
Hugging those lost
Within dreams our hearts blend.

Stirring, whirring,

picture blurring

Tossing, turning,

heart yearning

May I stay…?
just a bit longer.

Just for fun.

96

Incandescent

Too many nights spent
Under the warmth of incandescent bulbs
The moon and stars too beautiful to be forgotten
Lie dimmed in the overcrowded sky

Too many nights spent
Under bright fluorescent lights
Phosphorescent life illuminates ever so briefly
Much livelier in the night

By the warmth and brightness of your light
May it continue to allow our mortal eyes to see

97

Keys to Success

There truly is just a few keys to a healthy life
But they seem to be ever so hard to accomplish .

We often over complicate what we need to be doing.
Keep it simple.

1. Eat healthy
2. Exercise
3. Get a good night's sleep
4. Don’t smoke
5. Don't drink too much

While there are no guarantees in life, these can most definitely better your odds.

There are a few things to consider when pursuing a healthy life.
But why are they so difficult to do??

Eat your fruits and veggies
Walk, jog, run
Get your 8 hours
Stop smoking!
Limit the alcohol

Still looking for advice…
Well, the best thing you can do is

Eat a varied diet
Keep moving
Put down the phone and get to sleep!
Put the cancer sticks down!
Just a taste of wine, not the bottle!

Just listen.
Do these and you should do fine.

But if you need more then…

BONUS
Smile and laugh
Don't get too comfortable
Challenge yourself
Dream
Think
Do.

98

Nothing Here

What'd you expect?

99

A Break from the Chaos

Life is full of chaos

And I wouldn't have it any other way.

But sometimes, just sometimes

I need a break.

Goodbye for now...

100

100 Words

One Hundred words
Not all great
Perhaps they will collaborate

A little here, a little there
Searching far and wide
For these words to come alive

Today, tomorrow, another year
Meticulously scavenging
Frantically ravaging

Sometimes, more is less and less is more
In which I must confess
I'd prefer to write much, much less

Yet, May these words sing
Both far and wide
May these words come alive

If I had one hundred words...
which I do
I would spend them all with you

Alas, our time
It comes to end
I hope by now, I may call you friend.

Farewell for now.

- T.L. Larson

The journey continues. Life goes on. As much as I wish for it to stop and wait for me to catch up.

This book is dedicated to my father, but my special thanks will go to my daughters Aria and Layla. They are now my light and motivation. Thank you for all that you are and all that you will be. I look forward to seeing you grow and learn.

And to you the reader, thank you!

Thank you for taking the time to read this book!
I truly hope you found something you connected with and enjoyed.

If you indeed did enjoy this one, keep an eye out for part 3 to come out sometime in the next 9 years! Haha, we will see if I can push up this deadline. But currently it may be up to my little bosses. Take up any complaints with them please.

A Break from the Chaos has literally been my break from the chaos. It is my safe space to come and vent, breathe, and place random thoughts.
It is and has been a constant work in progress. I expect I will release another volume or two, depending on how well the writing spirit keeps up.

Made in the USA
Monee, IL
04 November 2026

67375757R00059